FATTY LIVER DIET FOOD LIST FOR BEGINNERS AND NEWLY DIAGNOSED

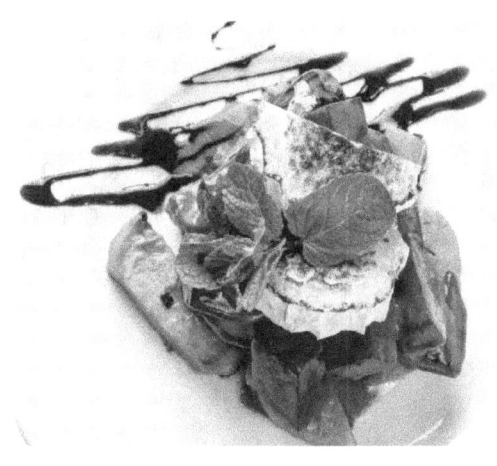

2 In 1 guide on what to eat for fatty healthy liver diet

Felicia O. Pace

To explore additional evidence-based and approved nutrition books similar to this one, please feel free to visit my Amazon store

https://author.amazon.com/books

Table of Contents

INTRODUCTION

Fatty liver disease, also known as hepatic steatosis, is a condition characterized by the accumulation of fat in liver cells. It is a growing health concern worldwide, often associated with lifestyle factors such as poor dietary choices, sedentary behavior, and obesity. The good news is that adopting a well-balanced and targeted diet can play a crucial role in managing and even reversing fatty liver disease. For beginners and those recently diagnosed, understanding the principles of a fatty liver diet is essential for promoting liver health and overall well-being.

What is a Fatty Liver Diet?

A fatty liver diet focuses on making dietary choices that reduce the burden on the liver and promote its healing. It aims to address the underlying causes of hepatic steatosis, such as insulin resistance, inflammation, and oxidative stress. The key principles of a fatty liver diet involve:

Balanced Macronutrients:
1. Prioritize a balanced intake of carbohydrates, proteins, and fats.

2. Choose complex carbohydrates over simple sugars to manage blood glucose levels.
3. Incorporate lean proteins and healthy fats while moderating overall calorie intake.

Healthy Fats:
1. Opt for unsaturated fats found in olive oil, avocados, nuts, and fatty fish.
2. Limit saturated and trans fats found in processed foods, red meat, and fried items.
3. Consider omega-3 fatty acids from sources like flaxseeds and fatty fish for their anti-inflammatory properties.

Complex Carbohydrates:
1. Choose whole grains, legumes, and fiber-rich foods to support stable blood sugar levels.
2. Minimize refined carbohydrates, sugary snacks, and beverages to reduce excess calorie intake.

Lean Proteins:
1. Prioritize lean protein sources such as poultry, fish, tofu, and legumes.
2. Limit consumption of red and processed meats that may contribute to inflammation.

Portion Control:
1. Practice mindful eating and control portion sizes to maintain a healthy weight.
2. Avoid overeating and listen to your body's hunger and fullness cues.

Hydration:
1. Stay well-hydrated with water and herbal teas.
2. Limit the consumption of sugary drinks and excessive caffeine.

Nutrient-Rich Foods:
1. Include a variety of fruits, vegetables, and antioxidant-rich foods to support liver health.
2. Emphasize foods containing vitamins and minerals like vitamin E, vitamin C, and selenium.

Getting Started with Your Fatty Liver Diet

Consult with a Healthcare Professional:
- Seek guidance from a healthcare professional or a registered dietitian for personalized advice based on your specific health needs and conditions.

Gradual Changes:

1. Introduce dietary changes gradually to make the transition more sustainable.
2. Focus on creating a well-rounded and enjoyable eating plan that aligns with your lifestyle.

Educate Yourself:
1. Learn about the nutritional content of foods, read labels, and make informed choices.
2. Understand the impact of dietary choices on liver health.

Regular Monitoring:
1. Regularly monitor your progress with healthcare professionals.
2. Adjust your diet based on feedback and changing health needs.

Lifestyle Modifications:
1. Complement your dietary changes with a healthy lifestyle, including regular physical activity and stress management.
2. Adopting a fatty liver diet is a positive step towards improving liver function and overall health. Remember, the goal is not only to manage the condition but to enhance your well-being for the long term. By embracing these dietary principles and making informed choices, you can take control of your health and

support your liver on the journey to recovery.

DIETARY GUIDELINES FOR MEAL PLANNING TIPS

Dietary guidelines for meal planning are crucial for managing fatty liver disease. Here are comprehensive meal planning tips for beginners and those newly diagnosed with fatty liver:

1. Balanced Macronutrients:
    1. Include a balance of carbohydrates, proteins, and fats in each meal.
    2. Prioritize complex carbohydrates like whole grains, fruits, and vegetables.
    3. Choose lean protein sources such as poultry, fish, tofu, and legumes.
    4. Opt for healthy fats found in olive oil, avocados, and nuts.

2. Portion Control:
    1. Practice portion control to avoid overeating and maintain a healthy weight.

2. Use smaller plates and bowls to manage portion sizes effectively.
3. Listen to your body's hunger and fullness cues.

3. Limit Added Sugars:
1. Minimize the intake of sugary beverages, sweets, and processed foods.
2. Check food labels for hidden sugars and opt for natural sweeteners when needed.

4. Choose Whole Foods:
1. Emphasize whole, minimally processed foods over refined and processed options.
2. Select whole grains, fresh fruits, vegetables, and unprocessed proteins.

5. Fiber-Rich Foods:
1. Include fiber-rich foods to support digestion and blood sugar control.
2. Choose whole grains, legumes, fruits, and vegetables regularly.

6. Hydrate Wisely:
1. Stay hydrated with water, herbal teas, and other non-caloric beverages.
2. Limit the consumption of sugary drinks and excessive caffeine.

7. Healthy Cooking Methods:

1. Opt for cooking methods such as baking, grilling, steaming, or sautéing.
2. Minimize frying and using excessive amounts of cooking oils.

8. Moderate Alcohol Consumption:
   1. If you consume alcohol, do so in moderation.
   2. Limit alcohol intake to recommended guidelines or as advised by your healthcare provider.

9. Include Omega-3 Fatty Acids:
   1. Incorporate sources of omega-3 fatty acids, such as fatty fish (salmon, mackerel), flaxseeds, and chia seeds.

10. Vitamin and Mineral-Rich Foods:
   2. Include foods rich in vitamin E (almonds, sunflower seeds), vitamin C (citrus fruits), and selenium (Brazil nuts).
   3. Consume a variety of colorful fruits and vegetables for a spectrum of nutrients.

11. Limit Saturated and Trans Fats:
   1. Minimize the intake of saturated fats found in red meat, full-fat dairy, and processed foods.
   2. Avoid trans fats often present in fried and commercially baked goods.

12. Meal Timing:
   1. Aim for regular meal times to maintain stable blood sugar levels.
   2. Include smaller, balanced meals throughout the day.

13. Consider Low-Glycemic Index Foods:
   a. Choose low-glycemic index foods to help manage blood sugar levels.
   b. Include options like whole grains, legumes, and non-starchy vegetables.

14. Limit Salt Intake:
   a. Control sodium intake by reducing the use of table salt and avoiding high-sodium processed foods.
   b. Choose herbs and spices for flavoring.

15. Consult with a Healthcare Professional:
   a. Seek guidance from a healthcare professional or a registered dietitian for personalized advice.
   b. Regularly monitor and adjust your diet based on your health progress.

Foods to avoid or Limit for fatty Fatty Liver Diet for Beginners and Newly Diagnosed

When following a fatty liver diet, it's crucial to identify and limit certain foods that may contribute to the progression of the condition. Here's a list of foods to avoid or limit for beginners and those newly diagnosed with fatty liver disease:

1. Added Sugars:
    1. Avoid: Sugary beverages, sodas, energy drinks, and sweetened fruit juices.
    2. Limit: Sweets, candies, pastries, and processed foods with high sugar content.

2. Highly Processed Foods:

1. Avoid: Processed snacks, fast food, and pre-packaged convenience foods.
2. Limit: Frozen meals and foods with additives and preservatives.

3. Saturated and Trans Fats:
    1. Avoid: High-fat red meats, full-fat dairy products, and fried foods.
    2. Limit: Processed foods with hydrogenated oils and commercially baked goods.

4. Excessive Salt:
    1. Avoid: High-sodium processed foods, canned soups, and salty snacks.
    2. Limit: Added salt in cooking; opt for herbs and spices for flavor.

5. Alcohol:
    1. Avoid: Excessive alcohol consumption can exacerbate liver damage.
    2. Limit: If you choose to consume alcohol, do so in moderation as advised by healthcare professionals.

6. White Bread and Refined Grains:
    1. Avoid: White bread, white rice, and other refined grains.
    2. Limit: Replace with whole grains like brown rice, quinoa, and whole wheat.

7. High-Fructose Corn Syrup:
    1. Avoid: Processed foods containing high-fructose corn syrup.
    2. Limit: Check food labels for hidden sources of added sugars.

8. Fried Foods:
    1. Avoid: Deep-fried foods, such as French fries and fried chicken.
    2. Limit: Choose healthier cooking methods like baking, grilling, or sautéing.

9. Processed Meats:
    1. Avoid: Sausages, hot dogs, bacon, and other processed meats.
    2. Limit: Choose lean cuts of fresh meat and poultry.

10. Highly Caffeinated Beverages:
    1. Avoid: Excessive consumption of coffee and energy drinks.
    2. Limit: Opt for moderate amounts of caffeine; consider herbal teas and water.

11. High-Calorie Snacks:
    1. Avoid: Chips, cookies, and other high-calorie snacks.
    2. Limit: Choose healthier snack options like nuts, seeds, and fresh fruits.

12. Artificial Sweeteners:
    1. Avoid: Products containing artificial sweeteners.
    2. Limit: Be cautious with diet sodas and sugar-free products.

13. High-Glycemic Index Foods:
    1. Limit: Foods that rapidly increase blood sugar levels, such as white potatoes and sugary cereals.

14. Unhealthy Cooking Oils:
    2. Avoid: Oils high in saturated fats, like palm oil and coconut oil.
    3. Limit: Opt for healthier cooking oils like olive oil.

15. Large Meals Late at Night:
    1. Avoid: Heavy meals close to bedtime.
    2. Limit: Opt for smaller, well-balanced dinners earlier in the evening.

Fruits and vegetables

Broccoli:
Calories: 55 per cup (chopped)
Fat: 0.6g
Sugar: 2.5g

Spinach:
Calories: 7 per cup (raw)
Fat: 0.1g
Sugar: 0.1g

Kale:
Calories: 33 per cup (chopped)
Fat: 0.5g
Sugar: 0.6g

Berries (Blueberries, Strawberries, Raspberries):
Calories: 50-85 per cup (varies by type)
Fat: 0.5-1g
Sugar: 7-15g

Avocado:
Calories: 240 per cup (sliced)
Fat: 21g

Sugar: 0.7g
Sweet Potatoes:
Calories: 180 per cup (mashed)
Fat: 0.2g
Sugar: 6.6g

Carrots:
Calories: 52 per cup (chopped)
Fat: 0.3g
Sugar: 6g

Beets:
Calories: 59 per cup (cooked)
Fat: 0.2g
Sugar: 9.2g

Grapes:
Calories: 104 per cup
Fat: 0.2g
Sugar: 23g

Cabbage:
Calories: 22 per cup (shredded)
Fat: 0.1g
Sugar: 1.5g

Tomatoes:
Calories: 32 per cup (chopped)
Fat: 0.4g
Sugar: 6.3g

Bell Peppers:
Calories: 46 per cup (chopped)
Fat: 0.5g
Sugar: 6g

Cauliflower:
Calories: 27 per cup (chopped)
Fat: 0.3g
Sugar: 2.5g

Oranges:
Calories: 62 per medium orange
Fat: 0.2g
Sugar: 12g

Brussels Sprouts:
Calories: 38 per cup (cooked)
Fat: 0.3g
Sugar: 1.9g

Whole grains

Quinoa:
Calories: 222 per cup (cooked)
Fat: 4g
Fiber: 5g

Brown Rice:
Calories: 215 per cup (cooked)
Fat: 1.8g
Fiber: 3.5g

Oats:
Calories: 147 per cup (cooked)
Fat: 2.5g
Fiber: 4g

Barley:
Calories: 193 per cup (cooked)
Fat: 0.7g
Fiber: 6g

Whole Wheat Pasta:
Calories: 174 per cup (cooked)
Fat: 1.3g
Fiber: 6g

Bulgur:
Calories: 151 per cup (cooked)
Fat: 0.4g
Fiber: 8g

Farro:
Calories: 337 per cup (cooked)
Fat: 1.7g
Fiber: 5.3g

Millet:
Calories: 207 per cup (cooked)
Fat: 1.7g
Fiber: 2.3g

Wild Rice:
Calories: 166 per cup (cooked)
Fat: 0.6g
Fiber: 3g

Buckwheat:
Calories: 155 per cup (cooked)
Fat: 1.5g
Fiber: 4.5g

Freekeh:
Calories: 329 per cup (cooked)
Fat: 2.2g
Fiber: 9.6g

Sorghum:
Calories: 143 per cup (cooked)
Fat: 1.5g
Fiber: 6.7g

Spelt:
Calories: 246 per cup (cooked)
Fat: 1.3g
Fiber: 10.7g

Teff:
Calories: 255 per cup (cooked)
Fat: 2.6g
Fiber: 10.6g

Amaranth:
Calories: 251 per cup (cooked)
Fat: 3.9g
Fiber: 9.3g

Lean protein

Chicken Breast (skinless, boneless):
Calories: 165 per 3.5 ounces (cooked)
Fat: 3.6g
Protein: 31g

Turkey (lean ground):
Calories: 170 per 3.5 ounces (cooked)
Fat: 8g
Protein: 22g

Fish (e.g., Salmon, Mackerel, Trout):
Calories: 206 per 3.5 ounces (cooked)
Fat: 13g
Protein: 22g

Tuna (canned in water):
Calories: 179 per 3.5 ounces (drained)
Fat: 1g
Protein: 40g

Shrimp:
Calories: 85 per 3.5 ounces (cooked)
Fat: 1.7g
Protein: 18g

Lean Beef (e.g., Sirloin, Tenderloin):
Calories: 250 per 3.5 ounces (cooked)
Fat: 17g
Protein: 26g

Pork Loin:
Calories: 143 per 3.5 ounces (cooked)
Fat: 3g
Protein: 25g

Eggs:
Calories: 68 per large egg (boiled)
Fat: 4.8g
Protein: 5.5g

Greek Yogurt (non-fat):
Calories: 100 per 6 ounces
Fat: 0g
Protein: 15g

Cottage Cheese (low-fat):
Calories: 206 per cup
Fat: 4.5g
Protein: 28g

Tofu:
Calories: 144 per cup (firm)
Fat: 8g
Protein: 16g

Lentils:
Calories: 230 per cup (cooked)
Fat: 0.8g
Protein: 17.9g

Chickpeas (Garbanzo Beans):
Calories: 269 per cup (cooked)
Fat: 4.2g
Protein: 14.5g

Skinless Turkey or Chicken Sausages:
Calories: 150 per 3.5 ounces (cooked)
Fat: 7g
Protein: 18g

Low-Fat Dairy (e.g., Milk, Cheese):
Calories: Varies (check packaging)
Fat: Varies (check packaging)
Protein: Varies (check packaging)

Healthy fats

Avocado:
Calories: 160 per avocado
Total Fat: 14.7g
Monounsaturated Fat: 10.5g

Olive Oil:
Calories: 120 per tablespoon
Total Fat: 14g
Monounsaturated Fat: 10g

Walnuts:
Calories: 185 per ounce (about 14 halves)
Total Fat: 18.5g
Omega-3 Fatty Acids: 2.6g

Chia Seeds:
Calories: 138 per ounce
Total Fat: 9g
Omega-3 Fatty Acids: 4.9g

Flaxseeds:
Calories: 150 per ounce
Total Fat: 12g
Omega-3 Fatty Acids: 6.4g

Salmon:
Calories: 206 per 3.5 ounces (cooked)
Total Fat: 13g
Omega-3 Fatty Acids: 2.3g

Almonds:
Calories: 160 per ounce (about 23 almonds)
Total Fat: 14g
Monounsaturated Fat: 8.8g

Coconut Oil:
Calories: 120 per tablespoon
Total Fat: 14g
Saturated Fat: 12g

Hemp Seeds:
Calories: 166 per ounce
Total Fat: 14.6g
Omega-3 Fatty Acids: 2.7g

Pistachios:
Calories: 156 per ounce (about 49 kernels)
Total Fat: 12.7g
Monounsaturated Fat: 6.6g

Dark Chocolate (70-85% cocoa):
Calories: 170 per ounce
Total Fat: 12g
Monounsaturated Fat: 7g

Sunflower Seeds:
Calories: 165 per ounce
Total Fat: 14.5g
Monounsaturated Fat: 3.2g

Olives:
Calories: 4 per medium-sized olive
Total Fat: 0.4g
Monounsaturated Fat: 0.3g

Pumpkin Seeds:
Calories: 151 per ounce
Total Fat: 13g
Monounsaturated Fat: 5.7g

Sardines:
Calories: 191 per 3.5 ounces (canned in oil)
Total Fat: 11g
Omega-3 Fatty Acids: 1.5g

Dairy:

Greek Yogurt (non-fat):
Calories: 100 per 6 ounces
Total Fat: 0g
Protein: 15g

Skim Milk:
Calories: 83 per cup
Total Fat: 0.2g
Protein: 8g

Low-Fat Cottage Cheese:
Calories: 206 per cup
Total Fat: 4.5g
Protein: 28g

String Cheese (part-skim):
Calories: 80 per piece
Total Fat: 6g
Protein: 7g

Low-Fat Plain Yogurt:
Calories: 154 per cup
Total Fat: 4g
Protein: 13g

Dairy Alternatives:

Almond Milk (unsweetened):
Calories: 13 per cup
Total Fat: 1g
Protein: 1g

Soy Milk (unsweetened):
Calories: 80 per cup
Total Fat: 4g
Protein: 7g

Coconut Milk (unsweetened):
Calories: 50 per cup
Total Fat: 4.5g
Protein: 0.5g

Oat Milk (unsweetened):
Calories: 80 per cup
Total Fat: 1.5g
Protein: 3g

Rice Milk (unsweetened):
Calories: 120 per cup
Total Fat: 2.5g
Protein: 1g

Cashew Milk (unsweetened):

Calories: 25 per cup
Total Fat: 2g
Protein: 0g
Hemp Milk (unsweetened):
Calories: 70 per cup
Total Fat: 5g
Protein: 2g

Flax Milk (unsweetened):
Calories: 25 per cup
Total Fat: 2.5g
Protein: 0g

Low-Fat or Unsweetened Coconut Yogurt:
Calories: Varies (check packaging)
Total Fat: Varies (check packaging)
Protein: Varies (check packaging)

Low-Fat Soy Yogurt:
Calories: Varies (check packaging)
Total Fat: Varies (check packaging)
Protein: Varies (check packaging)

Beverages

Water:
Calories: 0
Fat: 0g
No added sugars

Green Tea:
Calories: 0
Fat: 0g
No added sugars

Herbal Tea (unsweetened):
Calories: 0
Fat: 0g
No added sugars

Black Coffee (unsweetened):
Calories: 2 per 8 ounces
Fat: 0.2g
No added sugars

Sparkling Water (unsweetened):
Calories: 0
Fat: 0g
No added sugars

Vegetable Juice (low-sodium):
Calories: 50 per cup
Fat: 0.5g

Sugar: 10g
Lemon Water:
Calories: 0
Fat: 0g
No added sugars

Coconut Water (unsweetened):
Calories: 46 per cup
Fat: 0.5g
Sugar: 6.3g

Almond Milk (unsweetened):
Calories: 13 per cup
Fat: 1g
Protein: 1g

Soy Milk (unsweetened):
Calories: 80 per cup
Fat: 4g
Protein: 7g

Tomato Juice (low-sodium):
Calories: 41 per cup
Fat: 0.2g
Sugar: 9g

Hibiscus Tea (unsweetened):
Calories: 0
Fat: 0g
No added sugars

Ginger Tea (unsweetened):
Calories: 0
Fat: 0g
No added sugars

Cucumber Infused Water:
Calories: 0
Fat: 0g
No added sugars

Skim Milk:
Calories: 83 per cup
Fat: 0.2g
Protein: 8g

Herbs and Spices

Basil:
Calories: 1 per tablespoon
Fat: 0g

Cilantro (Coriander):
Calories: 0 per tablespoon
Fat: 0g

Parsley:
Calories: 1 per tablespoon

Fat: 0g

Oregano:
Calories: 3 per tablespoon
Fat: 0g

Thyme:
Calories: 3 per tablespoon
Fat: 0g

Rosemary:
Calories: 2 per tablespoon
Fat: 0g

Mint:
Calories: 2 per tablespoon
Fat: 0g

Turmeric:
Calories: 6 per tablespoon
Fat: 0.3g

Cinnamon:
Calories: 6 per tablespoon
Fat: 0.1g

Ginger:
Calories: 5 per tablespoon
Fat: 0.1g

Garlic (fresh or powdered):
Calories: 5 per tablespoon (powdered)
Fat: 0g
Chives:
Calories: 1 per tablespoon
Fat: 0g

Dill:
Calories: 2 per tablespoon
Fat: 0g

Paprika:
Calories: 6 per tablespoon
Fat: 0.3g

Chili Powder:
Calories: 6 per tablespoon
Fat: 0.3g

Legumes

Lentils:
Calories: 230 per cup (cooked)
Fat: 0.8g
Protein: 17.9g
Fiber: 15.6g

Chickpeas (Garbanzo Beans):

Calories: 269 per cup (cooked)
Fat: 4.2g
Protein: 14.5g
Fiber: 12.5g

Black Beans:
Calories: 227 per cup (cooked)
Fat: 0.9g
Protein: 15.2g
Fiber: 15g

Kidney Beans:
Calories: 225 per cup (cooked)
Fat: 0.9g
Protein: 15.4g
Fiber: 11.3g

Pinto Beans:
Calories: 245 per cup (cooked)
Fat: 1.1g
Protein: 15.4g
Fiber: 15.4g

Black-eyed Peas:
Calories: 160 per cup (cooked)
Fat: 0.5g
Protein: 5.2g
Fiber: 8.2g

Split Peas:

Calories: 231 per cup (cooked)
Fat: 0.8g
Protein: 16.4g
Fiber: 16.3g

Edamame:
Calories: 188 per cup (cooked)
Fat: 8g
Protein: 18.5g
Fiber: 8g

Cannellini Beans:
Calories: 225 per cup (cooked)
Fat: 0.9g
Protein: 15.3g
Fiber: 13.1g

Adzuki Beans:
Calories: 294 per cup (cooked)
Fat: 0.2g
Protein: 17.3g
Fiber: 17.4g

Navy Beans:
Calories: 255 per cup (cooked)
Fat: 0.9g
Protein: 15g
Fiber: 19g

Mung Beans:
Calories: 212 per cup (cooked)
Fat: 0.8g
Protein: 14.2g
Fiber: 15.4g

Butter Beans (Lima Beans):
Calories: 209 per cup (cooked)
Fat: 0.7g
Protein: 11.6g
Fiber: 13.2g

Chana Dal (Split Chickpeas):
Calories: 160 per cup (cooked)
Fat: 2.6g
Protein: 7.3g
Fiber: 8.4g

Red Lentils:
Calories: 230 per cup (cooked)
Fat: 0.4g
Protein: 17.9g
Fiber: 15.6g

Seafood

Salmon (wild-caught):
Calories: 206 per 3.5 ounces (cooked)
Total Fat: 13g
Omega-3 Fatty Acids: 2.3g
Protein: 22g

Mackerel:
Calories: 205 per 3.5 ounces (cooked)
Total Fat: 13g
Omega-3 Fatty Acids: 4.6g
Protein: 22g

Trout:
Calories: 148 per 3.5 ounces (cooked)
Total Fat: 6.9g
Omega-3 Fatty Acids: 1.5g
Protein: 20g

Sardines (canned in oil):
Calories: 191 per 3.5 ounces
Total Fat: 11g
Omega-3 Fatty Acids: 1.5g
Protein: 21g

Albacore Tuna (canned in water):
Calories: 128 per 3.5 ounces (drained)
Total Fat: 1.1g
Omega-3 Fatty Acids: 0.9g
Protein: 29g

Shrimp:
Calories: 85 per 3.5 ounces (cooked)
Total Fat: 1.7g
Protein: 18g

Cod:
Calories: 82 per 3.5 ounces (cooked)
Total Fat: 0.7g
Omega-3 Fatty Acids: 0.2g
Protein: 18g

Haddock:
Calories: 88 per 3.5 ounces (cooked)
Total Fat: 0.6g
Omega-3 Fatty Acids: 0.2g
Protein: 19g

Halibut:
Calories: 110 per 3.5 ounces (cooked)
Total Fat: 2.3g
Omega-3 Fatty Acids: 0.4g
Protein: 21g

Scallops:
Calories: 95 per 3.5 ounces (cooked)
Total Fat: 0.6g
Omega-3 Fatty Acids: 0.1g
Protein: 19g

Crab (blue crab):
Calories: 84 per 3.5 ounces (cooked)
Total Fat: 1.1g
Omega-3 Fatty Acids: 0.3g
Protein: 18g

Clams:
Calories: 74 per 3.5 ounces (cooked)
Total Fat: 1.3g
Omega-3 Fatty Acids: 0.2g
Protein: 14g

Lobster:
Calories: 89 per 3.5 ounces (cooked)
Total Fat: 0.9g
Omega-3 Fatty Acids: 0.2g
Protein: 18g

Oysters:
Calories: 68 per 3.5 ounces (cooked)
Total Fat: 2.2g
Omega-3 Fatty Acids: 0.2g

Protein: 8g

Tilapia:
Calories: 94 per 3.5 ounces (cooked)
Total Fat: 2.3g
Omega-3 Fatty Acids: 0.1g
Protein: 20g

Sweeteners

Natural Sweeteners:
Honey:
Calories: 64 per tablespoon
Total Fat: 0g

Maple Syrup (100% pure):
Calories: 52 per tablespoon
Total Fat: 0g

Agave Nectar:
Calories: 60 per tablespoon
Total Fat: 0g

Stevia (natural, unprocessed):
Calories: 0
Total Fat: 0g

Artificial Sweeteners:

Sucralose (Splenda):
Calories: 0
Total Fat: 0g
Aspartame (Equal, NutraSweet):
Calories: 0
Total Fat: 0g

Saccharin (Sweet'N Low):
Calories: 0
Total Fat: 0g

Acesulfame Potassium (Sunett, Sweet One):
Calories: 0
Total Fat: 0g

Monk Fruit Sweetener:
Calories: 0
Total Fat: 0g

Sugar Alcohols:

Xylitol:
Calories: 9.6 per teaspoon
Total Fat: 0g

Erythritol:
Calories: 0.2 per gram (about 6 calories per teaspoon)

Total Fat: 0g

Sorbitol:
Calories: 5.6 per teaspoon
Total Fat: 0g
Mannitol:
Calories: 1.5 per gram (about 4.5 calories per teaspoon)
Total Fat: 0g

Other Low-Calorie Sweeteners:

Allulose:
Calories: 0.4 per gram (about 1.2 calories per teaspoon)
Total Fat: 0g

Tagatose:
Calories: 1.5 per gram (about 4.5 calories per teaspoon)
Total Fat: 0g

HEALTHY AND EASY FOOD RECIPES

Breakfast

Oatmeal with Berries:
Calories: 150 per cup (cooked)
Total Fat: 3g
Fiber: 4g
Protein: 6g

Greek Yogurt Parfait with Nuts and Fruits:
Calories: 200 per cup (non-fat yogurt)
Total Fat: 10g
Protein: 20g
Fiber: 3g

Avocado Toast on Whole Grain Bread:
Calories: 200 per slice
Total Fat: 10g
Protein: 5g
Fiber: 5g

Chia Seed Pudding with Almond Milk:
Calories: 150 per 2 tablespoons (chia seeds)
Total Fat: 9g
Protein: 5g
Fiber: 8g

Egg White Omelet with Vegetables:
Calories: 150 per 3 large egg whites
Total Fat: 0g
Protein: 18g

Smoothie with Spinach, Banana, and Almond Milk:
Calories: 150 per cup
Total Fat: 3g
Protein: 5g
Fiber: 4g

Whole Grain Pancakes with Berries:
Calories: 200 per two 4-inch pancakes
Total Fat: 2g
Protein: 6g
Fiber: 3g

Cottage Cheese and Pineapple Bowl:
Calories: 200 per cup (low-fat cottage cheese)
Total Fat: 4g
Protein: 28g
Fiber: 2g

Quinoa Breakfast Bowl with Fruit and Nuts:
Calories: 250 per cup (cooked quinoa)
Total Fat: 5g
Protein: 8g

Fiber: 5g

Whole Grain Waffle with Greek Yogurt and Berries:
Calories: 180 per waffle
Total Fat: 6g
Protein: 8g
Fiber: 3g

Smoked Salmon on Whole Grain Bagel:
Calories: 300 per bagel
Total Fat: 6g
Protein: 15g
Fiber: 4g

Brown Rice Cake with Almond Butter and Banana Slices:
Calories: 200 per rice cake
Total Fat: 9g
Protein: 4g
Fiber: 4g

Fruit Salad with Walnuts:
Calories: 150 per cup
Total Fat: 9g
Protein: 2g
Fiber: 4g

Low-Fat Yogurt with Granola and Mixed Berries:
Calories: 250 per cup
Total Fat: 4g
Protein: 10g
Fiber: 5g

Peanut Butter Banana Smoothie:
Calories: 250 per cup
Total Fat: 12g
Protein: 8g
Fiber: 5g

Lunch

Grilled Chicken Salad:
Calories: 300 per serving (3 ounces of chicken)
Total Fat: 10g
Protein: 25g
Fiber: 4g

Quinoa and Vegetable Bowl:
Calories: 250 per cup (cooked quinoa)
Total Fat: 6g
Protein: 8g
Fiber: 5g

Baked Salmon with Steamed Broccoli:
Calories: 300 per serving (3.5 ounces of salmon)
Total Fat: 15g
Protein: 25g
Fiber: 3g

Turkey and Avocado Wrap on Whole Wheat Tortilla:
Calories: 350 per wrap
Total Fat: 15g
Protein: 20g
Fiber: 6g

Vegetable Stir-Fry with Tofu:
Calories: 250 per cup (tofu and mixed vegetables)
Total Fat: 10g
Protein: 15g
Fiber: 6g

Spinach and Feta Stuffed Chicken Breast:
Calories: 280 per serving (4 ounces of chicken)
Total Fat: 10g
Protein: 30g
Fiber: 2g

Black Bean and Vegetable Burrito Bowl:

Calories: 300 per bowl
Total Fat: 8g
Protein: 15g
Fiber: 10g

Chickpea Salad with Cucumber and Tomatoes:
Calories: 200 per cup
Total Fat: 8g
Protein: 7g
Fiber: 6g

Mushroom and Spinach Quiche (Crustless):
Calories: 180 per serving
Total Fat: 10g
Protein: 15g
Fiber: 2g

Sweet Potato and Lentil Curry:
Calories: 280 per cup
Total Fat: 5g
Protein: 10g
Fiber: 8g

Shrimp and Vegetable Skewers:
Calories: 250 per serving (4 ounces of shrimp)
Total Fat: 10g
Protein: 25g
Fiber: 3g

Whole Wheat Pasta with Tomato and Basil Sauce:
Calories: 300 per cup (cooked pasta)
Total Fat: 2g
Protein: 8g
Fiber: 6g

Lentil Soup:
Calories: 200 per cup
Total Fat: 2g
Protein: 10g
Fiber: 8g

Grilled Veggie Wrap with Hummus:
Calories: 300 per wrap
Total Fat: 10g
Protein: 10g
Fiber: 8g

Chicken and Vegetable Brown Rice Bowl:
Calories: 350 per bowl
Total Fat: 8g
Protein: 20g
Fiber: 5g

Dinner

Grilled Salmon with Roasted Vegetables:
Calories: 350 per serving (3.5 ounces of salmon)
Total Fat: 18g
Protein: 25g
Fiber: 5g

Turkey and Vegetable Stir-Fry:
Calories: 300 per serving (4 ounces of turkey)
Total Fat: 10g
Protein: 20g
Fiber: 8g

Baked Cod with Quinoa and Steamed Broccoli:
Calories: 320 per serving (3.5 ounces of cod)
Total Fat: 6g
Protein: 25g
Fiber: 6g

Chickpea and Spinach Curry:
Calories: 300 per serving
Total Fat: 10g
Protein: 12g
Fiber: 8g

Grilled Chicken Breast with Sweet Potato Mash:
Calories: 350 per serving (4 ounces of chicken)
Total Fat: 8g
Protein: 30g
Fiber: 6g

Vegetarian Chili with Black Beans and Quinoa:
Calories: 280 per serving
Total Fat: 5g
Protein: 12g
Fiber: 10g

Cauliflower Rice Stir-Fry with Tofu:
Calories: 250 per serving
Total Fat: 12g
Protein: 15g
Fiber: 8g

Lemon Garlic Shrimp with Brown Rice:
Calories: 320 per serving (4 ounces of shrimp)
Total Fat: 8g
Protein: 20g
Fiber: 4g

Grilled Vegetable and Quinoa Stuffed Peppers:
Calories: 280 per serving

Total Fat: 8g
Protein: 10g
Fiber: 8g

Chicken and Broccoli Quiche (Crustless):
Calories: 300 per serving
Total Fat: 15g
Protein: 25g
Fiber: 3g

Eggplant Parmesan with Whole Wheat Pasta:
Calories: 350 per serving
Total Fat: 10g
Protein: 15g
Fiber: 8g

Grilled Tofu Skewers with Vegetable Medley:
Calories: 280 per serving
Total Fat: 15g
Protein: 15g
Fiber: 6g

Salmon and Asparagus Foil Packets:
Calories: 300 per serving (3.5 ounces of salmon)
Total Fat: 15g
Protein: 25g
Fiber: 4g

Mushroom and Spinach Stuffed Chicken Breast:

Calories: 320 per serving (4 ounces of chicken)
Total Fat: 15g
Protein: 30g
Fiber: 2g

Black Bean and Corn Salad with Grilled Chicken:
Calories: 320 per serving (4 ounces of chicken)
Total Fat: 12g
Protein: 25g
Fiber: 8g

Snacks and Desserts

Snacks:

Greek Yogurt with Berries:
Calories: 150 per cup (non-fat yogurt)
Total Fat: 0g
Protein: 20g
Fiber: 3g

Hummus with Carrot Sticks:
Calories: 100 per 2 tablespoons (hummus)
Total Fat: 6g
Protein: 2g
Fiber: 3g

Almonds (unsalted):

Calories: 160 per ounce
Total Fat: 14g
Protein: 6g
Fiber: 3.5g

Apple Slices with Peanut Butter:
Calories: 200 per medium apple with 2 tablespoons of peanut butter
Total Fat: 12g
Protein: 6g
Fiber: 5g

Whole Grain Crackers with Cheese:
Calories: 150 per serving (6 whole grain crackers with 1 ounce of cheese)
Total Fat: 8g
Protein: 6g
Fiber: 3g

Cherry Tomatoes with Mozzarella Balls:
Calories: 120 per cup
Total Fat: 9g
Protein: 6g
Fiber: 2g

Rice Cakes with Avocado:
Calories: 150 per serving (2 rice cakes with half an avocado)
Total Fat: 12g
Protein: 2g
Fiber: 5g

Cucumber Slices with Tzatziki:
Calories: 50 per 1/2 cup (tzatziki)
Total Fat: 3g
Protein: 2g
Fiber: 1g

Desserts:

Dark Chocolate Covered Strawberries:
Calories: 100 per 3 strawberries
Total Fat: 5g
Protein: 1g
Fiber: 3g

Baked Apples with Cinnamon:
Calories: 120 per medium apple
Total Fat: 0.5g
Protein: 0.5g
Fiber: 5g

Yogurt Parfait with Granola and Berries:
Calories: 200 per serving
Total Fat: 5g
Protein: 8g

Fiber: 4g

Chia Seed Pudding with Mango:
Calories: 150 per 1/2 cup
Total Fat: 8g
Protein: 4g
Fiber: 8g

Frozen Banana Bites:
Calories: 50 per 2 pieces
Total Fat: 2g
Protein: 1g
Fiber: 1g

Berries with Whipped Cream:
Calories: 100 per cup (mixed berries with 2 tablespoons of whipped cream)
Total Fat: 7g
Protein: 1g
Fiber: 6g

Peach and Yogurt Popsicles:
Calories: 70 per popsicle
Total Fat: 2g
Protein: 3g
Fiber: 1g

Smoothies

Berry Blast:
Ingredients: Mixed berries, Greek yogurt, spinach, almond milk.
Calories: 200 per serving
Total Fat: 5g
Protein: 12g
Fiber: 7g

Green Dream:
Ingredients: Spinach, banana, avocado, pineapple, coconut water.
Calories: 250 per serving
Total Fat: 9g
Protein: 5g
Fiber: 8g

Tropical Paradise:
Ingredients: Mango, banana, Greek yogurt, orange juice.
Calories: 220 per serving
Total Fat: 3g

Protein: 9g
Fiber: 4g

Citrus Delight:
Ingredients: Orange, kiwi, pineapple, plain yogurt, chia seeds.
Calories: 180 per serving
Total Fat: 3g
Protein: 6g
Fiber: 8g

Peanut Butter Banana Protein Smoothie:
Ingredients: Banana, peanut butter, Greek yogurt, almond milk.
Calories: 300 per serving
Total Fat: 15g
Protein: 18g
Fiber: 5g

Detox Green Smoothie:
Ingredients: Kale, cucumber, green apple, lemon, coconut water.
Calories: 120 per serving
Total Fat: 1g
Protein: 3g

Fiber: 5g

Blueberry Bliss:
Ingredients: Blueberries, spinach, banana, flaxseeds, coconut milk.
Calories: 180 per serving
Total Fat: 6g
Protein: 4g
Fiber: 6g

Chocolate Avocado Smoothie:
Ingredients: Avocado, cocoa powder, banana, almond milk.
Calories: 250 per serving
Total Fat: 15g
Protein: 5g
Fiber: 8g

Cherry Almond Smoothie:
Ingredients: Cherries, almond butter, Greek yogurt, water.
Calories: 220 per serving
Total Fat: 10g
Protein: 10g
Fiber: 5g

Minty Pineapple Cucumber Smoothie:
Ingredients: Pineapple, cucumber, mint leaves, lime, coconut water.
Calories: 150 per serving
Total Fat: 1g

Protein: 3g
Fiber: 4g

Strawberry Banana Oatmeal Smoothie:
Ingredients: Strawberries, banana, oats, almond milk.
Calories: 230 per serving
Total Fat: 4g
Protein: 6g
Fiber: 7g

Peachy Keen:
Ingredients: Peaches, Greek yogurt, honey, ice cubes.
Calories: 190 per serving
Total Fat: 2g
Protein: 8g
Fiber: 3g

Carrot Cake Smoothie:
Ingredients: Carrots, banana, cinnamon, nutmeg, almond milk.
Calories: 200 per serving
Total Fat: 5g
Protein: 4g
Fiber: 6g

Raspberry Coconut Refresher:
Ingredients: Raspberries, coconut water, coconut flakes, Greek yogurt.
Calories: 160 per serving

Total Fat: 6g
Protein: 5g
Fiber: 8g

Vanilla Almond Protein Shake:
Ingredients: Almond milk, vanilla protein powder, banana, almond butter.
Calories: 280 per serving
Total Fat: 12g
Protein: 18g
Fiber: 4g

SHOPPING LIST

Fresh Produce:
1. Spinach
2. Kale
3. Broccoli
4. Cauliflower
5. Brussels sprouts
6. Asparagus
7. Carrots
8. Bell peppers
9. Cucumbers
10. Zucchini
11. Tomatoes
12. Avocado
13. Berries (blueberries, strawberries, raspberries)
14. Apples

15. Oranges
16. Lemons
17. Lime
18. Mango
19. Pineapple
20. Grapes
21. Watermelon
22. Peaches
23. Cherries
24. Pears
25. Bananas

Whole Grains:
1. Quinoa
2. Brown rice
3. Oats (steel-cut or rolled)
4. Whole wheat pasta
5. Barley
6. Farro
7. Bulgur
8. Whole grain bread
9. Whole grain tortillas

Lean Proteins:
1. Salmon (wild-caught)
2. Mackerel
3. Trout
4. Cod
5. Tuna (canned in water)

6. Skinless chicken breast
7. Turkey breast
8. Lean cuts of beef or pork
9. Tofu
10. Tempeh
11. Eggs
12. Greek yogurt (non-fat or low-fat)
13. Cottage cheese (low-fat)

Legumes:
1. Black beans
2. Chickpeas
3. Lentils
4. Kidney beans
5. Pinto beans
6. Edamame

Nuts and Seeds:
1. Almonds
2. Walnuts
3. Flaxseeds
4. Chia seeds
5. Pumpkin seeds
6. Sunflower seeds

Dairy and Dairy Alternatives:
1. Low-fat or non-fat milk
2. Low-fat or non-fat yogurt
3. Unsweetened almond milk
4. Unsweetened coconut milk

Healthy Fats:
1. Olive oil (extra virgin)
2. Avocado oil
3. Flaxseed oil
4. Coconut oil
5. Avocados

Herbs and Spices:
1. Turmeric
2. Ginger
3. Garlic
4. Cinnamon
5. Basil
6. Parsley
7. Cilantro
8. Rosemary
9. Thyme

Seafood:
1. Shrimp
2. Crab
3. Clams
4. Oysters
5. Scallops
6. Lobster

Beverages:
1. Green tea
2. Herbal tea

3. Water (stay well-hydrated)
4. Coconut water

Whole Wheat and Grain Products:
1. Whole wheat flour
2. Whole grain cereal
3. Whole grain crackers
4. Whole grain tortilla chips

Sweeteners:
1. Honey
2. Maple syrup
3. Stevia

Frozen Foods:
1. Frozen berries
2. Frozen vegetables
3. Frozen fish fillets
4. Veggie burgers (low in saturated fat)

Condiments:
1. Mustard
2. Balsamic vinegar

CONCLUSION

In conclusion, adopting a fatty liver diet for beginners and those newly diagnosed is a proactive and empowering step towards managing and potentially reversing this common liver condition. The dietary principles outlined provide a roadmap for making informed choices that support liver health and overall well-being.

Understanding the impact of balanced macronutrients, healthy fats, lean proteins, and fiber-rich foods is fundamental to crafting meals that nourish the body without overburdening the liver. By emphasizing whole, minimally processed foods and incorporating nutrient-dense choices, individuals can positively influence liver function and contribute to an improved quality of life.

Limiting or avoiding foods high in added sugars, saturated and trans fats, as well as processed and fried items, plays a pivotal role in reducing the strain on the liver. Likewise, moderating alcohol intake, opting for whole grains, and being mindful of portion sizes contribute to a comprehensive approach to managing fatty liver disease.

As individuals embark on this dietary journey, it is crucial to recognize that progress is gradual, and sustainable changes are key. The journey to improved liver health is not just about restriction; it is about embracing a diverse and colorful array of foods that not only nurture the liver but also delight the palate.

Consulting with healthcare professionals or registered dietitians ensures personalized guidance tailored to individual health needs. Regular monitoring, lifestyle modifications, and a commitment to long-term well-being are integral aspects of managing fatty liver disease.

In essence, the fatty liver diet for beginners and newly diagnosed individuals is a positive lifestyle transformation that extends beyond managing a health condition—it is a holistic approach to nurturing the body, fostering habits that promote vitality, and embarking on a journey towards a healthier, more vibrant life.

Dear Cherished Readers

I trust this book has served as a wellspring of inspiration, solace, and valuable insights for you. Each recipe was crafted with love, meticulous attention to detail, and a profound understanding of effective utilization ensuring wholesome and nutritious meals.

Your reviews, experiences, and insights are invaluable. Every evaluation propels me to enhance and tailor my work to better cater to your needs. Let's engage in a meaningful discussion—a dialogue that transcends the written words, forging a deeper connection. Your thoughts are the driving force behind continuous improvement.

Warm regards,

Felicia O. Pace

To explore additional evidence-based and approved nutrition books similar to this one, please feel free to visit my Amazon store

https://author.amazon.com/books